Ana Isabel Correia
Libânia Araújo

Cervical Cancer Prevention

Ana Isabel Correia
Libânia Araújo

Cervical Cancer Prevention

Gynaecology

ScienciaScripts

Imprint

Any brand names and product names mentioned in this book are subject to trademark, brand or patent protection and are trademarks or registered trademarks of their respective holders. The use of brand names, product names, common names, trade names, product descriptions etc. even without a particular marking in this work is in no way to be construed to mean that such names may be regarded as unrestricted in respect of trademark and brand protection legislation and could thus be used by anyone.

Cover image: www.ingimage.com

This book is a translation from the original published under ISBN 978-3-330-19720-6.

Publisher:
Sciencia Scripts
is a trademark of
Dodo Books Indian Ocean Ltd. and OmniScriptum S.R.L publishing group

120 High Road, East Finchley, London, N2 9ED, United Kingdom
Str. Armeneasca 28/1, office 1, Chisinau MD-2012, Republic of Moldova, Europe
Printed at: see last page
ISBN: 978-620-8-23607-6

Summary

Objectives: The aim of this review is to address the issue of cervical cancer prevention through a bibliographical survey of existing publications, so that it can become an auxiliary tool for updating and improving clinical practice.

Data sources: PubMed database, RORENO and GLOBOCAN data and specialized textbook.

Review methods: Of the 639 articles obtained, 46 were selected by reading the title and abstract, which responded to the objective of this review, as well as other studies that allowed a general approach to this topic.

Results: Cervical cancer is a major public health problem worldwide. It is one of the most common cancers, both in terms of incidence and mortality, and ranks first in many developing countries. Cervical infection with oncogenic HPV subtypes is a major etiological factor in cervical cancer. This factor is necessary for the development of high-risk lesions and cancer, but there are others. More than 100 genotypes have been identified, of which around 40 preferentially infect the genital organs. Around 70% of cervical cancer cases are due to HPV types 16 and 18, these being high-risk subtypes. Secondary prevention strategies, through screening, should be associated with primary prevention, through education and vaccination, which are complementary forms of prevention. There are two commercial vaccines against HPV,

Gardasil® and Cervarix®, which are prophylactic vaccines and have no therapeutic efficacy. Secondary prevention is based on the detection of lesions by cytology, immunological recognition and colposcopy, integrated into organized and opportunistic screening programmes. The combination of these strategies increases the effectiveness of any program to combat cervical cancer.

Conclusions: Much remains to be done in the field of CC prevention, both in terms of education, vaccination and screening.

Keywords: Cervical neoplasms/prevention & control ; Papillomavirus infections ; Papillomavirus vaccines; Cervical cancer screening.

Article Type: Review

Index

1 Introduction

Cervical cancer (CCU) is a major public health problem worldwide.[1]

Statistically, it is the second most common cancer in the world.[2,3] It is one of the most common cancers, both in terms of incidence and mortality, and ranks first in many developing countries.[1-6]

It is estimated that around 500,000 cases are detected every year worldwide and that more than 2,500,000 deaths occur.[4,6-9] It is estimated that every two minutes there is a woman affected by CC, so this problem seems to be bigger than that of acquired immunodeficiency syndrome (AIDS).[10]

Cervical infection by the human papilloma virus (HPV) is the main etiologic factor in CC and has been shown to be its precursor in more than 99% of cases.[11]

Thus, the prevention of HPV infection has a major impact on the incidence of CC and primary and secondary prevention strategies are crucial in addressing this important public health problem.

The aim of this monograph is a general approach to the subject of CC prevention, through a bibliographical review of existing publications, so that it can be an auxiliary tool for updating and improving clinical practice.

2 Methods

On October 23, 2010, a PubMed search was carried out with the following search equation: (("uterine cervical neoplasms"[MeSH Terms] OR ("uterine"[All Fields] AND "cervical "[All Fields] AND "neoplasms" [All Fields]) OR "uterine cervical neoplasms" [All Fields] OR ("cervical" [All Fields] AND "cancer"[All Fields]) OR "cervical cancer"[All Fields]) AND ("prevention and control"[Subheading] OR ("prevention"[All Fields] AND "control "[All Fields]) OR "prevention and control "[All Fields] OR "prevention" [All Fields]). The search was limited to review articles from the last 5 years, with no language limit. A total of 639 articles were retrieved. From these reviews, 46 that corresponded to the aim of this monograph were selected by reading the title and abstract, as well as other studies that allowed a general approach to this topic.

In order to obtain epidemiological data on CC, on the recommendation of Dr. Libania Araujo, personal contact was made with Dr. Maria Josd Bento at the Epidemiology Department of the Portuguese Institute of Oncology (IPO) in Porto, who indicated the websites www.roreno.com.pt and www.iarc.fr where it was possible to find the most up-to-date information on the subject. Dr. Maria Josd Bento also provided the book -Cancer Epidemiology and Prevention!, which is included in the bibliography for this monograph.

3 Results

A. Some thoughts on Cervical Cancer

A1. Incidence and Mortality

According to the Global Cancer Estimates (GLOBOCAN), the incidence of CC in the world in 2008 was 529828 (age-standardized rate per 100000 (ASR(W)) 15.3) and mortality 275128 (ASR(W)) 7.8).[3]

In general terms, it is much more common in developing countries, where 83% of cases occur, and where CC constitutes 15% of female cancers, with a risk before the age of 65 of 1.5%. In developed countries, CC is responsible for 3.6% of new cancers, with a cumulative risk of 0.8%.[2] Less developed countries have the highest burden in terms of morbidity and mortality, largely due to the lack of organized screening programs.[12]

The highest incidence rates are observed in Sub-Saharan Africa, Malaysia, Latin America and the Caribbean, Central Asia and Southeast Asia. Incidence rates are generally low in developed countries. Age-standardized rates are lower than 14.5/100000. This pattern is relatively recent, however, before the introduction of screening programs in 1960-1970, the incidence in most countries in Europe, North America, and Australia/New Zealand was similar to those in developing countries today. Very low rates are also observed in China (6.8/100,000 inhabitants) and West Asia (5.8/100,000), with the lowest recorded rate being 0.4/100,000 in Ardabil, in northwestern Iran.[2]

Mortality rates are substantially lower than incidence rates. The mortality coefficient for incidence is 55% worldwide. Survival varies from region to region and the prognosis is better in low-risk regions. Even in developing countries, where cases of advanced cancer appear, the survival rate was reasonable (an estimated 44% age-adjusted survival rate versus 61% in developed areas). In general, over the years there has been a decline in mortality and incidence of CC, mainly in Western countries, due to well-developed screening programs, and this decline is also evident in some developing countries.[2]

According to GLOBOCAN, in 2008, 60,951 new cases of In Portugal, the incidence of CC was 949 (ASR(W) 12.2) and the mortality 346 (ASR (W) 3.6).[3]

According to data from the Northern Regional Cancer Registry (RORENO), CC had an incidence of 15.3/100,000 and was the sixth most common cancer in 2005, affecting 4.5% of women, with a mortality/incidence

ratio of 27%.[13]

A2. Risk factors

Cervical infection with oncogenic HPV subtypes is the major etiologic factor in CC, and is extremely common compared to the development of CC, which is relatively rare. This indicates that additional etiological factors are involved in the evolution of lesions, including sociodemographic and behavioral factors, variability in the host's immune response, genetic and familial susceptibility, smoking, parity and other gynecological and obstetric events, use of oral contraceptives, co-infection with other bacterial or viral agents, occupational factors and probably diet.[1,2,14-16]

A3. Pathogenesis

The development of CC includes three fundamental stages: HPV infection, progression of the infection to cancerous lesions and invasion.[4]

HPV is transmitted sexually, and in most cases infections are transient, asymptomatic and clinically insignificant, and may not result in microscopic or macroscopically evident lesions.[1,15,17]

HPV is a deoxyribonucleic acid (DNA) virus with around 8,000 base pairs and a viral capsid made up of two proteins, L1 and L2. More than 100 HPV genotypes have been identified, of which around 40 preferentially infect the genital organs: vulva, vagina, cervix, penis and perianal areas.[1,9,16,18-20]

The base cells are infected by the viruses, which arrive through microtraumas of the mucosa. Infection can develop in two ways: progressive episomal replication along the various layers of the malpighian epclium, until the virions are released on the surface of the mucosa by exfoliation of the superficial squamous cells, infecting neighboring cells; the viral genome integrates the cell genome and the E6 and E7 proto-oncogenes, initiating carcinogenesis.[18]

The E6 and E7 proteins have been shown to play a cooperative role in the transformation of proteins *in vitro*. E6 binds to and promotes the degradation of the tumor suppressor protein p53 by forming a complex that requires the molecular protein E6-AP. In addition, the E6 protein activates telomerase. E7 is the main transforming protein and binds to and inactivates the retinoblastoma tumor suppressor protein.[1,20,21]

HPV infection is very common, but in most cases it is transient and self-limiting. In 80% of cases, it resolves spontaneously after one to two years. The infection becomes persistent in the remaining 20%, a predisposing condition for an unfavorable evolution. In 3 to 4% of cases, it evolves into cervical intraepithelial neoplasia (CIN), of which 0.7 to 1% into CIN 2-3 (true precancerous lesion) and 0.1% into invasive cancer, with a variable progression time, usually around 15 years.

The viral origin of CC is well established. Several studies have shown that HPV DNA can be found in 99.7% of cervical cancers (squamous and adenocarcinomas), with types 16, 18, 45 and 31 being the most frequently found.[9,15,18,19,22] Theoretically, if HPV infection could be completely eradicated, most genital cancers could be prevented.[23]

Based on these observations, anogenital HPVs were divided into two groups: the first associated with the development of genital cancer was called high risk (HPV16, 18, 26, 31, 33, 35, 39, 45, 51, 52, 53, 56, 58, 59, 66, 68, 73, 82) and the second associated with benign lesions, with low oncogenic potential, called low risk HPVs (HPV 6, 11, 40, 42, 43, 44, 54, 61, 72, 81).[14,1824]

Around the world, 70% of SCC cases are due to HPV types 16 and 18 (type 16 is responsible for 54% and 18 for around 17%), with types 45, 31, 33 and 52 responsible for most of the remaining cases.[9,21] HPV types 6 and 11 are responsible for 90% of genital warts.[21]

Asymptomatic infections with both high-risk and naturally low-risk HPV types are the main sexually transmitted diseases: they are found in around 8-12% of all sexually active women.[7,16]

Currently, there is epidemiological, clinical and biochemical evidence that infection of the cervix with high-risk HPV types is a necessary factor for the development of the vast majority of cases of cervical cancer and high-grade lesions.[1,2,6,12,17,25]

B. Cervical Cancer Prevention

Preventive medicine actions are important procedures for preventing illnesses or diagnosing them in the early stages and guiding them towards the right treatment. Preventing illness is the most effective and economical way of maintaining health.

The peak prevalence of HPV in women is around 5 to 7 years after the start of sexual life. In contrast, the peak of screening for precancerous lesions is in women in the late third, early fourth decades of life, approximately 10 to 15 years after the start of sexual life, at ages when the prevalence of HPV decreases significantly.[4]

CC is a disease in which prevention can be effective at both primary and secondary levels, since its central etiology is infection by a well-defined virus. This prevention of virus infection has a major impact on the incidence of this cancer; and the development process takes around 10 to 20 years, giving the opportunity to interfere long before it develops.[6,17]

Secondary prevention strategies, through screening, should be associated with primary prevention, through education and vaccination, as complementary prevention strategies. This association improves the effectiveness of any program to combat CC. In order to reduce mortality from CC, it is extremely important to prevent HPV infection, diagnose it and treat it early and correctly.[26]

Challenges to guaranteeing the success of the prevention of this disease are the attitude of governments and policymakers, affordable prices, education at all levels, overcoming barriers to vaccination and continued adherence to screening programs.[12]

B1. Primary Prevention

Primary prevention of CC consists of preventing HPV infection.[4,6] It aims to reduce risk through behavioral attitudes towards sexual health and the use of vaccination against high-risk HPV.[8]

B1.a) Education

Health education aims to relate quality and commitment to life and not simply the absence of illness. In order to change the axis of the health/disease binomial, it is essential to stimulate attitudes and new procedures in the face of disease problems, so that health is seen as everyone's responsibility and not just a governmental responsibility.[15]

Numerous studies have shown that the general population's knowledge of HPV is very limited. That's why it's important to increase levels of knowledge on this subject, particularly by including it in the health education curriculum at school. In the context of health professionals, knowledge on the subject also varies between different groups, so they should be involved in training actions tailored to the needs of each group.[18]

Education should be aimed at patients of both sexes and should include information on primary prevention methods such as reducing the number of sexual partners and condom use.[17,27,28] Young people should be encouraged to talk about their doubts with their partner and take responsibility for sexual decisions once they have been informed and before they become sexually active. It should be borne in mind that more than half of HPV infections occur between the ages of 15 and 24. Therefore, young people should be educated about the following facts about HPV: genital HPV is usually transmitted through direct skin contact, most often during penetrative genital contact (anal or vaginal); women whose partners use latex condoms have lower rates of CC, however, condom use does not eliminate the risk of HPV transmission or 100% of sexually transmitted diseases. Young people should also be informed that the vaccination does not protect against all types of HPV that cause SCC and genital warts; it is not indicated for the treatment of SCC; it is not a live virus vaccine and does not contain viral DNA, so you can become infected from taking the vaccine; after the vaccine, women still need to have their regular screening.[27,28]

B1.b) Vaccination

HPV vaccines began to be studied about 10 years ago.[23] Highly effective HPV vaccines are now available, allowing new directions in the approach to CC. Vaccinating adolescents can reduce the average risk of contracting CC by around 44% if 70% coverage is achieved. A successful vaccination program has the potential to save hundreds of thousands of lives in several countries.[9]

There are two commercial HPV vaccines (Gardasil® and Cervarix®), one or both of which are currently approved in more than 100 countries around the world.[29] Both are produced using recombinant technology, consisting of self-assembling virus-like particles (VLPs), and have shown high immunogenicity.[7,24,30] VLPs are produced by cloning the main genes of the viral capsid of different HPV types and inserted into vectors. These VLPs are very similar to HPV virions and do not contain gendritic material, so they are neither infectious nor oncogenic. They induce high levels of neutralizing antibodies when administered intramuscularly, with rapid access of VLPs to blood vessels and lymph nodes. They are also potent activators of antigen-presenting cells.[18,20]

Due to their high immunogenicity, they are able to reduce a large proportion of cases of CC.[12] In addition, they have been shown to be highly effective in preventing persistent infections and lesions, not only of the cervix, but also of the anus, vagina and vulva.[7]

However, to be successful in terms of public health, they need to be widely implemented to the target population properly, preferably before the first sexual intercourse.[12]

Unfortunately, vaccines are still very expensive and inaccessible for many public health initiatives in developing countries.[30] They include two HPV types involved in the development of cancer (types 16 and 18) and therefore only partial protection against cancer can be expected (70/100), making it necessary to implement new strategies for the detection of precursor lesions and cancer in the post-vaccination era.[7,17,30] Therefore, after HPV vaccination, women still need to participate in CC screening programs.[31]

HPV vaccines have been shown to be effective (>90%) in preventing persistent HPV infections and precancerous lesions of target types, and for up to five years in women with serum HPV positivity.[4]

Vaccination can prevent the precursor changes of invasive cancer, as long as they are caused by the HPV types that are covered by the vaccination.[29]

In most individuals, HPV infection triggers a strong local cellular immune response, with eradication of the infection and significant protection (although not 100%) against subsequent infections with the same type of HPV.[18]

HPV vaccines are not therapeutic. The vaccine does not inhibit epithelial base cells already contaminated by HPV, which continue to transform epithelial layers into cervical dysplasia. There is hope among clinicians, already supported by initial data, that the vaccines will be able to neutralize HPV virions in host tissues from both self-inoculation infections and infections in organs other than the cervix, thus making it possible for these vaccines to prevent less common types of HPV associated with cancer of the penis, vagina, vulva, anus, oral cavity and oropharynx.[32]

Quadrivalent vaccine - Gardasil®

The Gardasil® quadrivalent vaccine was developed by Merck *& Co. Inc.* and approved in the United States, the European Union and other countries in 2006.[20]

This vaccine contains VLPs of HPV 16, 18, 6 and 11 purified and mixed with the amorphous adjuvant aluminum hydroxyphosphate sulfate, and inserted into vectors (yeast).[19,24]

The vaccination schedule used was an intramuscular dose of 0.5mL at 0, 2 and 6 months.14,30,33

The Gardasil® study program included around 27,000 volunteers (adolescents aged 9 to 15 and women aged 16 to 26) recruited in 33 countries on all continents.[18,30] The randomized, double-blind Phase III clinical trials conducted with the quadrivalent vaccine to assess efficacy involved around 18,000 women. After 2 years of follow-up, they showed 100% efficacy in cervical precancerous lesions (CIN 2-3 and cervical adenocarcinoma *in situ* (AIS)), vulvar lesions (VIN 2-3), vaginal lesions (ValN 2-3) and genital condylomas associated with HPV types 6, 11, 16 and 18. Published results at 5 years showed 96% efficacy in persistent infection and 100% in CIN 1-3 and condylomas related to HPV 6, 11, 16 and 18.[18,19] Trials are underway to evaluate the efficacy of the quadrivalent vaccine in men in terms of lesion prevention, as well as its impact on the transmission of infection.[18]

As for the safety of the vaccine, in the phase IIb studies the most frequent local adverse effects were erythema, pain and edema, but these did not exceed 10% compared to placebo. The most common systemic adverse effects were subfebrile temperature (10% with the vaccine vs 9% with placebo) and headache (19% with the vaccine vs 20% with placebo). There was no significant incidence of serious adverse effects, namely

bronchospasm.18,32,33

Some women became pregnant during the studies. Overall, 10.7% of the women became pregnant in the Gardasil® group and 12.6% in the placebo group. Among the women who became pregnant within 30 days of vaccination, there were five cases of congenital anomalies compared to zero in the placebo group, but none of these anomalies were related to the vaccination. On the other hand, in women whose pregnancy started more than 30 days after vaccination, there were 10 cases of anomalies in the vaccine group and 16 cases in the placebo group. A group of teratology experts concluded that these events were probably not associated with Gardasil® or its adjuvant. During the trials, 995 women breastfed (500 with the vaccine and 495 on placebo) with no vaccine-related adverse reactions in the breastfed infants or any disturbance in breastfeeding. The compatibility of the concomitant administration of Gardasil® with the Hepatitis B vaccine has been demonstrated.[18]

Bivalent vaccine - Cervarix ®

The bivalent Cervarix® vaccine was developed by *GlaxoSmithKline Biologicals* and approved in the European Union in 2007, as well as in other countries.[20]

This vaccine contains HPV 16 and 18 VLPs purified and mixed with aluminum hydroxide adjuvant and monophosphoryl lipid A, and inserted into vectors (baculovirus).[18,19,24]

The vaccination schedule used was an intramuscular dose of 0.5mL at 0, 1 and 6 months.[24,33]

A phase II, randomized, double-blind trial involving 1113 women aged 15 to 25 was carried out, followed by a new trial with 776 participants, to extend follow-up for a further 36 months. The results published after four and a half years are as follows: 100% efficacy in persistent HPV 16 and 18 infection; 100% protection for any degree of CIN. Phase III trials are underway, involving around 35,000 women from various countries.[18,34]

As for the safety of the vaccine, the results of phase IIb trials showed that the most frequent local adverse effects were erythema, pain and swelling at the injection site, but these did not exceed 5-9% compared to placebo. Systemic adverse effects such as headaches, fatigue, pruritus and gastrointestinal symptoms were seen in equal proportions in the placebo group and the vaccine group. Overall, 16.6% of those vaccinated and 13.6% of the placebo group had a temperature > 37.5°C. With regard to serious adverse effects, there was no increase in incidence in the vaccine group.[18,32]

Data on pregnancy and congenital malformations have not yet been published. It is important to carry out long-term surveillance studies to monitor the safety of vaccines and identify any rare adverse effects.[18]

Projecting the benefits of the two vaccines has been the subject of several published studies. If 100% coverage is considered, both vaccines can be expected to reduce the incidence of CC by 70 to 75%; CIN 2 and 3 by 50%; CIN 1 by 25%, in addition to reducing other carcinomas related to HPV 16 and 18. The quadrivalent vaccine can be expected to reduce CIN 1 by more than 10% and reduce the incidence of condylomas by 90%, as well as reducing other lesions related to HPV 6 and 11, such as laryngeal papillomatosis. The two HPV vaccines did not significantly modify the course of the disease in women with lesions at the time of vaccination, so they are not therapeutically effective.[18,35]

Duration of Immunity

As far as the duration of immunity is concerned, at 4-5 years of age, both vaccines maintain very high antibody levels (10 to 14 times higher than natural infection levels).[9,30,35] Effective immunogenicity is guaranteed and 100% efficacy is maintained at 53 months with the bivalent vaccine and at 60 months with the quadrivalent vaccine, in the prevention of cervical dysplasia caused by HPV 16 and HPV 18 and condylomas (in the case of the quadrivalent vaccine). Antibody titers after vaccination are higher than those induced by natural infection and seem to last longer, suggesting that the duration of protection with the vaccine may be longer. The duration of protection after vaccination is currently unknown and will be determined by long-term follow-up studies, which are currently underway. 18,35

Cross immunity

Trials of the bivalent vaccine showed partial protection against persistent infections with HPV types 31, 33, 52 and 45, with a 94.2% reduction in transient infections related to HPV 45 and a 54.5% reduction in those related to HPV 31.[18,34,35] Studies with the quadrivalent vaccine have shown protection against disease caused by HPV types 31, 33, 35, 52 and 58. However, cross-immunity is partial (59%). As already mentioned, HPV types 16 and 18 are responsible for 70% of CC cases. HPV types 31/33/35/45/52/56 are responsible for the remaining 20-30% of SCC cases. Thus, a polyvalent vaccine containing these 8 types of HPV can effectively protect against more than 90% of cases of SCC. ,[3335]

Vaccination age

Both vaccines induced high concentrations of specific antibodies to the four or two genotypes of VLPs they contain. The levels of antibodies induced are maximum at the end of the first month after the third dose of the vaccine and progressively fall until 18 months, stabilizing until 4-5 years - the maximum period of evaluation available. The immune response was maximum in the 9 to 15 year-old group, progressively decreasing with age, but always remaining significantly higher than that induced by natural infection.[18,33]

From a clinical point of view, the vaccines were 100% effective in preventing lesions related to HPV 16 and 18 in young women with no contact with HPV, regardless of age. Increasingly early sexual activity is a reality all over the world. In Portugal, a survey carried out by the Portuguese Society of Gynecology revealed that 49.6% of girls aged 15-19 had already started having sex. Several studies show that around 50% of women become infected with at least one type of HPV between 2 and 5 years after starting sexual activity. As HPV 16 and 18 are the most frequent genotypes in adolescents and young women, the maximum potential benefit of the vaccine will be achieved if it is administered before the onset of sexual activity.[9,18]

Based on the available scientific evidence, the *Food and Drug*

Administration (FDA) and the European Medical Agency (EMEA) have approved the quadrivalent vaccine for the group of women aged 9-26 years, considering adolescents before the start of sexual activity as the preferred target for vaccination.[18-20,24,32] The 11-13 age group is an excellent opportunity for vaccination, taking advantage of the comprehensive health examination recommended by the Directorate-General for Health for this age group.[36] Some studies propose that vaccination could benefit women over the age of 26 who have not previously been exposed to HPV 16 or 18 and those who may subsequently have new sexual partners. 12,16,30,36,37

B2. Secondary Prevention

Secondary prevention is a means of detecting carcinogenic HPV infection and treating women with precancerous lesions at an early stage.[4,6,8,38]

The three methods of detection are cytology, colposcopy and immunological recognition of the virus.[8]

In many developed countries that have organized screening programs, the incidence and mortality of CC have been reduced substantially.[38] Cytology screening has contributed to the substantial decline in CC in developed countries over the last five decades.[30] However, screening programs are inefficient in many regions of the world where the appropriate infrastructure is lacking.[30,38]

B2.a) Screening methods

Cytology

Cytology or the Pap test was validated and introduced in 1940.[5,20]

A strong correlation has been observed between the start of cytology screening and a reduction in the incidence of and mortality from CC. The effectiveness of cytology screening programs has been adequately demonstrated in countries such as Denmark, Finland, Iceland, Norway, Sweden and Colombia.[8]

Currently, Pap smear screening is essential for detecting the altered cells that can appear in women infected with HPV. By identifying these altered cells, screening aims to detect the disease when it is still at an undeveloped stage and can be treated, with fewer problems for the woman. Screening aims to prevent the disease from reaching the invasive stage, but it doesn't prevent previous cell changes. [39,40]

Colposcopy

When cytology is performed in conjunction with colposcopy, it has a negative predictive value of close to 100% for CC, which is why it is recommended by many schools.[41] With combined detection strategies, referral for colposcopy is much more frequent and the likelihood of a positive test having a high-grade lesion is substantially lower. [42]

Immunological Recognition

Worldwide interest in a potential HPV test in CC prevention programs is growing, both as a complement to the cytological screening approach and as the primary selection. This stems from two consistent observations. Firstly, HPV testing has an average of 25% higher sensitivity but around 10% lower specificity than cytology for detecting high-grade intraepithelial lesions (HSIL).[4,29,42,43] Secondly, the combination of cytology and the HPV test achieves a sensitivity and negative predictive value approaching 100%.[6,8,40]

B2.b) Types of Tracking

There are two types of screening, organized (population) and opportunistic, which are used in Europe. The two systems have different characteristics.[41,44]

Organized screening is a preventive medicine intervention, through the systematic application of a previously validated screening technique, which aims to reduce invasive carcinoma.

In an organized screening program, it is necessary to: define a target population (all sexually active women); administer the screening test to the target women at a specified interval (1-5 years); achieve a high level of screening coverage (> 70%); establish an effective call-back system for investigations; and treat women with serum positivity.[9]

A screening technique is not in itself a diagnostic technique. The ideal screening test must be reliable, sensitive, reproducible, convenient and low-cost. To have an impact on mortality, it must achieve a minimum coverage of 60% of the target population. The currently validated technique for population screening for CC is cytology. Its efficacy and effectiveness have been widely demonstrated in regions where it has been applied in a programmed, systematic and continuous manner.[41]

The HPV DNA detection test has been mentioned in numerous studies, also as a screening test. Its characteristics make it a useful test when combined with cytology or even as an initial and isolated screening test in women over 30. The immunological recognition of HPV as a screening test can detect approximately twice as many high-grade lesions as are detected by cytology. [45]

The recommendations for this type of screening are: start at the age of 25-64, interval cytology every 3 years after 2 satisfactory and negative annual results, and HPV test at the age of 35. If everything is negative, the screening interval is extended to 5 years. [41]

An organized HPV screening program has been proven to prevent 80% of deaths from CC. [45]

Opportunistic screening is when a woman undergoes cytology at a regular gynecological appointment. In this case, the diagnostic guarantees required by good medical practice should be offered.

Most cases of CC occur in unscreened women, so reaching these women is a priority objective. [41]

One of the great disadvantages of opportunistic screening is that it doesn't involve a significant number of the target population and often repeats cytologies excessively on low-risk women, increasing costs and without guaranteeing quality. [41]

The recommendations for this type of screening are: first cytology 3 years after the first sexual intercourse, repeated every 3 years; after 3 negative results, simultaneous cytology and colposcopy (optional); from the age of 35, HPV test (optional), if negative, repeat after 5 years. If the results are negative and there are no risk factors or changes in the couple's personal circumstances, it may be recommended to repeat the test every 3 years. The interval between tests should be shortened and the annual interval should be maintained when there are risk factors and in immunocompromised women.[40,41]

Opportunistic screening shows lower overall reductions in CC than organized screening programs; the effectiveness of screening can vary from one region to another; it tends to screen women from higher socio-economic groups who already access the health system regularly and have a lower risk of cervical cancer; it tends to screen some women more often than necessary; it doesn't screen women from lower socio-economic groups and minorities as necessary. For all these reasons, although opportunistic screening can reduce CC, it is less effective than organized screening and promotes health inequalities.[46]

The limited sensitivity of the techniques used for screening partly explains why cervical cancers continue to appear in populations with organized screening. However, when discussing the sensitivity of cytology, it is necessary to differentiate between the sensitivity of an isolated cytology and the sensitivity of a cytology screening program. Repeat cytology makes it possible to detect cases that have been missed.[41]

The ideal screening test should have, in addition to high sensitivity, a high positive predictive value and select only women with significant disease (CIN 2 -3 or cancer) or progression potential. However, both cytology and HPV DNA analysis detect an excess of women with positive or inconclusive results (atypical squamous cells of undetermined significance (ASC-US), low-grade squamous intraepithelial lesion (LSIL)), non-significant lesions that regress spontaneously. This leads to a high burden of care for their diagnosis and treatment, with increased anxiety for women.

In order to improve specificity and positive predictive value, new molecular markers that are indicators of significant disease or potential for progression are being investigated. The detection of HPV genome integration could be a useful parameter for assessing the risk of progression of intraepithelial lesions. Another parameter being investigated is the detection of active transcription of HPV oncogenes or the proteins resulting from their expression.[41]

4 Conclusions

CC is an extremely important pathology in women's health. Since this pathology is both preventable and curable, prevention strategies play a crucial role.

There is still a lot to be done in the field of CC prevention. Education, the basic strategy of primary prevention, needs greater investment. There are numerous studies showing that the general population's knowledge of HPV is very limited. That's why it's important to increase knowledge levels on this subject, both in schools and among health professionals and even the general population. Vaccination is the other primary prevention method with the potential to reduce the incidence and mortality of CC. In this field, measures are needed to promote vaccination and define the vaccination age in order to benefit as many women as possible. Studies on prophylactic vaccines are ongoing and require more time for definitive conclusions. The emergence of therapeutic vaccines will be a reality in the near future. Secondary prevention through screening methods needs greater investment, especially in developing countries, since screening has contributed to a substantial decline in CC in developed countries over the last five decades. Still under study are wet cytology and HPV-DNA detection as screening methods, in order to find the ideal screening test with optimized sensitivity and specificity.

It can therefore be concluded that the prevention of CC is crucial for controlling this important public health problem. Vaccination in conjunction with organized screening programs can theoretically prevent 100% of CC.

Thanks

I would like to thank Dr. Libania Araujo for her hard work, dedication and support in preparing this monograph. I would also like to thank Dr. Maria Joao Bento from the Epidemiology Department of the Portuguese Institute of Oncology in Porto, who kindly provided me with a bibliography containing the epidemiological data included in this monograph.

5 Bibliographical references

1. Schottenfeld D, Fraumeni J. Cancer Epidemiology and Prevention. 3rd ed. Oxford University Press; 2006. p. 1044-1064.

2. Parkin M, Bray F, Ferlay J, Pisani P. Global Cancer Statistics, 2002. CA Cancer Journal for Clinicians 2005;55:74-108.

3. GLOBOCAN 2008 (IARC): Cancer Incidence, Mortality and Prevalence Worldwide [database on the Internet]. IARC 2010 [accessed: 2010 Oct 23]; Available at: URL: http://globocan.iarc.fr/factsheets/cancers/cervix.asp.

4. Scarinci IC, Garcia FA, Kobetz E, Partridge EE, Brandt HM, Bell MC, et al. Cervical cancer prevention: new tools and old barriers. Cancer 2010 Jun 1;116(11):2531-42.

5. Safaeian M, Solomon D, Castle PE. Cervical cancer prevention-cervical screening: science in evolution. Obstet Gynecol Clin North Am 2007 Dec;34(4):739-60.

6. The prevention of cervical cancer in developing countries. BJOG: an International Journal of Obstetrics and Gynaecology 2005;112:1204-1212.

7. Madrid-Marina V, Torres-Poveda K, Lopez-Toledo G, Garcia-Carranca A. Advantages and disadvantages of current prophylactic vaccines

against HPV. Arch Med Res 2009 Aug;40(6):471-7.

8. Sehgal A, Singh V. Human papillomavirus (HPV) infection & screening strategies for cervical cancer. Indian J Med Res 2009 Sep;130(3):234-40.

9. Choudhury P. Preventing cervical cancer: pediatricians role. Indian Pediatr 2009 Mar;46(3):201-3.

10. Tjalma WA. Cervical cancer and prevention by vaccination: results from recent trials. Ann Oncol 2006 Sep;17(Suppl 10):217-23.

11. Montgomery K, Bloch JR. The human papillomavirus in women over 40: implications for practice and recommendations for screening. J Am Acad Nurse Pract 2010 Feb;22(2):92100.

12. Garland SM, Smith JS Human papillomavirus vaccines: current status and future prospects. Drugs 2010 Jun 18;70(9):1079-98.

13. Bento MJ. Northern Regional Oncology Registry (RORENO). Porto: Instituto Portugues de Oncologia do Porto; 2005 [access in: 2010 Oct 23]; Available at: URL: http://roreno.com.pt/images/stories/pdfs/roreno_05.pdf.

14. Irico G, Escobar H, Marinelli B. Cervical cancer prevention: an update. Rev Fac Cien Med Univ Nac Cordoba 2005;62(2 Suppl 1):37-47.

15. Cruz A, Monteiro C, Paula L, Reis A, Saddi A, Santos R. Human

pappilomavirus and public health: cervical cancer prevention. Ciencia & Saude Coletiva 2010;15 Suppl 1:10551060.

16.	Teitelman AM, Stringer M, Averbuch T, Witkoski A. Human papillomavirus, current vaccines, and cervical cancer prevention. J Obstet Gynecol Neonatal Nurs 2009 JanFeb;38(1):69-80.

17.	Denny L. Prevention of cervical cancer. Reprod Health Matters 2008 Nov;16(32):18- 31.

18.	Portuguese Society of Gynecology, Portuguese Section of Colposcopy and Cervico-Vulvovaginal Pathology, Portuguese Section of Oncological Gynecology. National consensus meeting - HPV vaccine 2007.

19.	Broomall EM, Reynolds SM, Jacobson RM. Epidemiology, clinical manifestations, and recent advances in vaccination against human papillomavirus. Postgrad Med 2010 Mar;122(2):121-9.

20.	Lowy DR, Solomon D, Hildesheim A, Schiller JT, Schiffman M. Human papillomavirus infection and the primary and secondary prevention of cervical cancer. Cancer 2008 Oct 1;113(7 Suppl):1980-93.

21.	Long HJ 3rd, Laack NN, Gostout BS. Prevention, diagnosis, and treatment of cervical cancer. Mayo Clin Proc 2007 Dec;82(12):1566-74.

22.	Schwartz LA. Cervical cancer: disease prevention and

informational support. Can Oncol Nurs J 2009 Winter-Spring;19(1):6-9.

23. Kawana K. HPV vaccine for cervical cancer prevention. Nippon Rinsho 2010 Jun;68 (6):1163-8.

24. Bhatla N, Joseph E. Cervical cancer prevention & the role of human papillomavirus vaccines in India. Indian J Med Res 2009 Sep;130(3):334-40.

25. Hrgovic Z, Izetbegovic S. Primary prevention of cervical carcinoma. Med Arh 2007;61(1):49-51.

26. Azam F, Shams-ul-Islam M. Prevention of human papilloma virus infection with vaccines. J Pak Med Assoc 2010 Aug;60(8):676-81.

27. Heavey E. Start early to prevent genital HPV infection-and cervical cancer. Nursing 2008 May;38(5):62-3.

28. Kollar LM, Kahn JA. Education about human papillomavirus and human papillomavirus vaccines in adolescents. Curr Opin Obstet Gynecol 2008 Oct;20(5):479- 83.

29. Franceschi S, Cuzick J, Herrero R, Dillner J, Wheeler CM. EUROGIN 2008 roadmap on cervical cancer prevention. Int J Cancer 2009 Nov 15;125(10):2246-55.

30. Sankaranarayanan R. HPV vaccination: the promise & problems. Indian J Med Res 2009 Sep;130(3):322-6.

31. Janssen PG, Boomsma LJ, Buis PA, Collette C, Boukes FS,

Goudswaard AN. Summary of the practice guideline 'Prevention and early diagnosis of cervical cancer' of the Dutch College of General Practitioners. Ned Tijdschr Geneeskd 2009;153:A517.

32.   Harper DM. Prevention of human papillomavirus infections and associated diseases by vaccination: a new hope for global public health. Public Health Genomics 2009;12(5- 6):319-30.

33.   D'Andrilli G, Bovicelli A, Giordano A. HPV vaccines: state of the art. J Cell Physiol 2010 Sep;224(3):601-4.

34.   Szarewski A. HPV vaccine: Cervarix. Expert Opin Biol Ther 2010 Mar;10(3):477-87.

35.   Stanley M. Human papillomavirus vaccines versus cervical cancer screening. Clin Oncol (R Coll Radiol) 2008 Aug;20(6):388-94.

36.   Wright TC Jr, Huh WK, Monk BJ, Smith JS, Ault K, Herzog TJ. Age considerations when vaccinating against HPV. Gynecol Oncol 2008 May;109(2 Suppl):S40-7.

37.   Simon P, Poppe W. Should the antipapillomavirus vaccination after the age of 25 be advised? J Gynecol Obstet Biol Reprod (Paris) 2008 Dec;37(8):748-52.

38.   Grce M. Primary and secondary prevention of cervical cancer. Expert Rev Mol Diagn 2009 Nov;9(8):851-7.

39.   Cuzick J, Arbyn M, Sankaranarayanan R, Tsu V, Ronco G,

Mayrand MH, et al. Overview of human papillomavirus-based and other novel options for cervical cancer screening in developed and developing countries. Vaccine 2008 Aug 19;26(10 Suppl):K29-41.

40.   Widdice LE, Moscicki AB. Updated guidelines for pap tests, colposcopy, and human papillomavirus testing in adolescents. J Adolesc Health 2008 Oct;43(4 Suppl):S41-51.

41.   Portuguese Society of Gynecology, Portuguese Section of Colposcopy and Cervico-Vulvovaginal Pathology. Consensus on Cervico-Vulvovaginal Pathology 2004.

42.   Ronco G, Giorgi Rossi P. New paradigms in cervical cancer prevention: opportunities and risks. BMC Womens Health 2008 Dec 17;8:23.

43.   Kinney W, Stoler MH, Castle PE. Special commentary: patient safety and the next generation of HPV DNA tests. Am J Clin Pathol 2010 Aug;134(2):193-9.

44.   Breitenecker G. Cervical cancer screening: past-present-future. Pathologe 2009 Dec;30(Suppl 2):128-35.

45.   Grce M, Davies P. Human papillomavirus testing for primary cervical cancer screening. Expert Rev Mol Diagn 2008 Sep;8(5):599-605.

46.   Everything about cervical cancer prevention. European Cervical

Cancer Association 2009 [accessed: 2010 Oct 23]; Available at: URL:

www.ecca.info/pt.

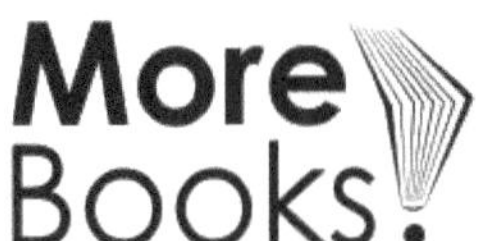

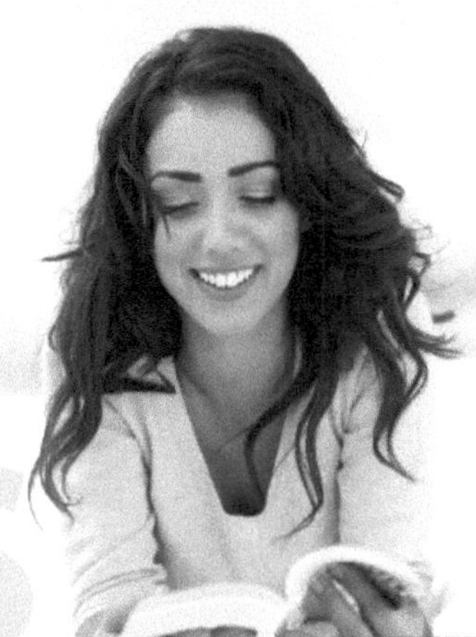

I want morebooks!

Buy your books fast and straightforward online - at one of world's fastest growing online book stores! Environmentally sound due to Print-on-Demand technologies.

Buy your books online at
www.morebooks.shop

Kaufen Sie Ihre Bücher schnell und unkompliziert online – auf einer der am schnellsten wachsenden Buchhandelsplattformen weltweit! Dank Print-On-Demand umwelt- und ressourcenschonend produziert.

Bücher schneller online kaufen
www.morebooks.shop

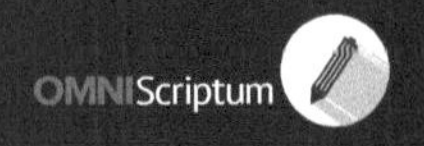

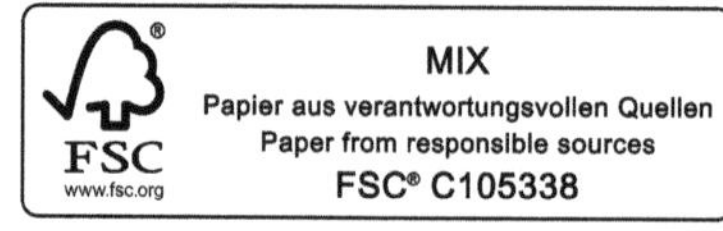

Printed by Books on Demand GmbH, Norderstedt / Germany